SLEEP WELL TONIGHT

simple ways to prevent sleeplessness

Barbara L. Heller

The mission of Storey Publishing is to serve our customers
by publishing practical information that encourages personal independence
in harmony with the environment.

Edited by Robin Catalano and Jennifer Travis Donnelly
Cover design by Wendy Palitz
Cover background illustrations by Alexandra Eckhardt
Cover image art © Juliette Borda
Herb illustrations on pages 30, 31, 33, 37, and 39 by Sarah Brill; those on
    pages 42 and 43 by Beverly Duncan
Text design and production by Susan Bernier

Storey books are available for special premium and promotional uses and for cus-
tomized editions. For further information, please call Storey's Custom Publishing
Department at 1-800-793-9396.

Printed in the United States by Lake Book
10 9 8 7 6 5 4 3 2

ISBN 1-58017-893-6

Table of Contents

Introduction • 1

The Facts of Sleep • 5

Self-Help Strategies for Sound Slumber • 8

Relaxation Techniques • 13

10 Ways to a Better Night's Sleep • 18

Herbal Therapy • 25

10 Herbs for Sleep and Relaxation • 28

How to Use Herbs for Sleep • 45

And Now, Good Night • 60

Introduction

How many hours a night do you sleep? Is your sleep deep and refreshing? Or do you find it hard to fall asleep, your mind racing with worries and thoughts from the day? Do you toss and turn, rouse often, and wake up tired? Or do you consistently wake too early? If you experience any of these symptoms, you are not alone.

One in three Americans doesn't get enough sleep. According to the National Sleep Foundation, two thirds of Americans report a recognizable sleep problem. The National Commission on Sleep Disorders asserts that "America is sleep-deprived with serious consequences."

Consider the following:

• Estimates suggest that 95 percent of those with sleep disorders go undiagnosed.

• Thirty-seven percent of Americans report being so sleepy during the day that it interferes with daily activities. This increases to 52 percent for shift workers.

• More than 5 billion doses of tranquilizers and sleeping pills are prescribed annually in the United States.

For most of us, sleep problems are temporary and are caused by stress, the demands of work, an impossibly long chore list, travel, or recuperation from illness. Some people, like shift workers and the parents of newborns, may experience longer periods of disturbed sleep. Aging can also affect the quality and quantity of our sleep.

What are the effects of all this sleeplessness? Tiredness correlates with decreased productivity and effectiveness, as well as irritability. You become unfocused and short-tempered, quick to project your ill humor onto others. In addition, fatigue can have tragic consequences. Drowsy drivers cause an estimated 100,000 car crashes yearly, many with fatal results. Everything from crises at nuclear power plants to train wrecks have been attributed to the poor judgment of overtired workers.

How Do You Get Help?

Although sleeplessness takes many forms, there are two levels of sleep problems. One is the persistent, serious, long-term inability to get a good night's sleep. The first step in getting help for this is a visit to your healthcare practitioner, who may refer you to a sleep clinic. Sleep disorders, when not properly diagnosed, are serious and potentially dangerous. For example, snorers and overweight sleepers are prone to sleep apnea, a breath-stopping disorder that increases the risk of heart attack, stroke, and death. Tests done at sleep clinics can identify sleep problems, including apnea, and provide treatment.

The other level of sleep problems is occasional or periodic insomnia. Almost everyone goes through a period when getting a good night's sleep is difficult. Sleep can be disturbed in three major ways: You can have difficulty falling asleep, be unable to remain asleep through the night, and wake too early to function well.

For those of us with this level of sleep disturbance, there are many natural alternatives to sleepless nights and sleeping pills. This book provides practical, safe, and simple home remedies to help you relax naturally and sleep better. You can choose sleep-inducing strategies and relaxation techniques, or you can try changing your sleep habits and attitudes. Or you may want to try herbal aids, including calming medicinal teas and tinctures, soothing baths, and sleep pillows.

Relax and enjoy!
Here's to your sound slumber.

The Facts of Sleep

Sleep is essential to our physical and emotional health. Each night, every 90 minutes, we cycle through five different levels of sleep. We experience many physiological changes, including muscle contractions and relaxations as well as alterations in temperature, blood pressure, and pulse. During periods of deeper sleep, our bodies repair and heal themselves. In other phases, sleep is shallower, our bodies still, but our brains are more active. The increased brain activity of the REM (rapid eye movement) period helps consolidate our daily memories and signifies that we are dreaming. Most sleep researchers agree that dreaming is a creative process that can be healing and emotionally soothing.

How Much Sleep Do You Need?

The simplest answer to this question is that you need enough sleep to feel alert when you are awake. Every individual is different, but the average person needs 7 to 8 hours of sleep to function well. Most of us get somewhere between 5 and 10 hours, but nearly one third of Americans get by on 6 hours or less.

In the past, people lived more in tune with the cycles of natural sunlight. In 1910 the average American clocked in more sleep than her contemporary counterpart: nine hours a night. Many researchers think we should return to the natural patterns of the past, rising with the sun and going to sleep soon after sunset.

Do You Have a Sleep Problem?

Do you dread facing the day after a sleepless night? Are you dragging in the morning or losing steam too early? Do you start to doze after dinner in front of the TV? Are you generally irritable or forgetful? Does your boss, spouse, or friend comment on your grumpiness or low energy level?

Look at the facts and figures of your sleep habits. Do you routinely sleep seven hours per night or less? Would you like to sleep more if you "just could find the time"? How you feel during the day and the feedback you get from others about your mood or performance are two keys to assessing a sleep problem.

If you are sleeping poorly, a physical exam can help identify medical conditions and medications that are known sleep-thieves. Insomnia can be a secondary effect of heart disease, diabetes, chronic sinus infections, depression, gastroesophageal reflux, and a host of other conditions. Certain drugs prescribed for allergy relief, asthma, and heart conditions, as well as several painkillers, antidepressants, and antihistamines, can contribute to sleeplessness. Talk with your healthcare practitioner about the possibility of changing your medication or the dose or time you take it.

Keeping a Sleep Diary

The best way to start getting more sleep is to keep track of your sleep patterns and your level of satisfaction with the quantity and quality of your slumber. This assessment can help you choose possible remedies for refreshing sleep and can be valuable to a healthcare practitioner if self-help strategies are not potent enough. See the box at right for questions to ask yourself about your sleep patterns.

Self-Help Strategies for Sound Slumber

What can you do to ensure fewer sleepless nights and more refreshing rest? After assessing your sleep habits and patterns, you must first address any specific mental or physical concerns. Have a checkup if you have any questions about your condition. Identifying and treating the underlying cause of insomnia are paramount.

The goal is to reestablish refreshing, nonmedicated sleep. Many self-help strategies can help you achieve this.

Personal Sleep Assessment Questions

1. What time did you go to bed last night?

2. About how long did it take you to fall asleep?

3. Did you awaken during the night? If so, how many times? What did you do when you awoke (stay in bed, go to the bathroom, have a cigarette, clean, worry, and so on)? How long did it take you to get back to sleep?

4. How many hours did you sleep last night, in total?

5. What time did you get up in the morning?

6. Did you use an alarm clock?

7. On a scale of 1 (still tired) to 5 (refreshed), how did you feel when you woke up?

8. On a scale of 1 (drowsy or fatigued) to 5 (energetic), how would you rate your functioning during the day?

9. How did you feel today? Were you anxious, depressed, irritable, forgetful, or accident-prone?

Enhancing Your Sleep Environment

Is your bedroom generally conducive to sound sleep? Is it comfortable, cozy, cool, and quiet enough? Is your mattress old or saggy? Perhaps it is time for a replacement, or you may need a new pillow.

Light levels in the room may affect how you fall asleep and awaken. Although a bright light may make for easier reading (no business tomes or thrillers before bed, though), overall room illumination should not be harsh. And remember, do not turn on the lights when you get up in the middle of the night. Doing so may trick your body into thinking it is morning and make it hard for you to get back to sleep. Use a night light or flashlight.

Is your bedroom used for activities unrelated to sleep? Is it a mini office? What you choose to do in the bedroom, and in bed, greatly influences how you sleep. In fact, many sleep clinics recommend that only two activities take place in bed: sleeping and sex.

If you suffer from allergies, they may be contributing to your sleep problems. Consult an allergist or healthcare professional about air filters and other methods of reducing dust mites, molds, pollens, and other airborne allergens in your sleep environment.

Even if you have been sleeping quite peacefully in your bedroom for years, changing the environment can help to break a recent sleep-difficulty pattern.

Increasing Your Physical Activity

Engaging in physical activity three to six hours before bedtime can help induce deeper and higher-quality sleep in two ways. First, during aerobic exercise our

 Timing Your Exercise

The timing of exercise is very important. Early-morning exercise may have many health benefits, but it does not seem to affect sleep ability or quality. On the other hand, exercising too close to bedtime can be stimulating, resulting in more sleep disturbances.

bodies release endorphins, naturally occurring antidepressants. Physiologically, these "feel-good" chemicals help us enjoy the time we are awake and experience more restful sleep. Second, movement earlier in the day helps to readjust our body temperature cycles. This adjustment causes the subtle evening temperature drop that is the body's cue to transition to slumber. A Stanford University study reported that 20 to 30 minutes of afternoon exercise significantly decreased the time it took insomniacs to fall asleep.

Nutritional Aids

Diet also affects the quality of sleep. Boosting your levels of B vitamins and ensuring that you get adequate calcium and magnesium — both natural relaxants — can help stop insomnia. Eating a small snack of complex carbohydrates like bread, pasta, or a baked potato within an hour of bedtime also may help your body chemistry slow down.

Relaxation Techniques

While most people equate nighttime relaxation with television, this isn't the best way to promote sleep if you're having trouble with insomnia. Instead, look to these all-natural, simple, soothing solutions, and make a habit of practicing them regularly.

Yoga

The practice of yoga, a Hindu health discipline, teaches physical and mental activities designed to strengthen muscles, build flexibility, increase energy, and encourage relaxation and spiritual development.

The basic postures, called *asanas,* are a series of stretches and breathing exercises that require no special equipment. Yoga can be done in a small amount of space almost anywhere, making it a perfect solution for the insomniac at home or on the road.

The best way to learn yoga is by taking a class with a qualified teacher. The feedback and hands-on instruction are keys to success. If local classes are not available, there are many books and tapes with easy-to-follow directions. Yoga anytime during the day is de-stressing. For the sleep deprived, I also recommend a 15- to 30-minute yoga session before bed to help unwind and to release the pressures of the day.

The Relaxation Response

No time or inclination to learn a new skill, especially now, when you are stressed and tired? There are some simple but profound techniques that you can begin using today.

The Relaxation Response, first described by Herbert Benson in his book of the same name, is an easy-to-learn, modified version of meditation. In looking for innovative ways to treat patients with high blood pressure, Benson and his Harvard University team distilled medical-scientific and spiritual writings from the East and West. The authors of

Relaxation Response Instructions

In a comfortable position, breathe fully and naturally. Pay attention to your breath. Silently repeat the word "one" as you breathe. Inhale, think "one"; exhale, take a breath in, focus on the word "one," and exhale. Continue for 10 to 20 minutes. For the greatest benefit, practice this once or twice daily.

Can't stop thinking when you try to sit quietly? Thoughts and distractions are normal. Observe the thoughts and let them pass. It is as if you are in a small boat gently gliding down a river, a peaceful trip without much effort. There are many people, animals, and objects of interest along the shore. You note them but don't try to become involved with any; soon they move out of your range of vision and consciousness. Allow your thoughts to take a similar voyage.

If you do get involved in an internal discussion, don't fight it. Acknowledge it and then return to the focus on your breath and the word one.

The technique may feel awkward the first few times. The challenge is to do it for at least 10 minutes once or twice a day for two weeks. Then you can evaluate your progress. Do you feel more relaxed? If so, stick with it. The benefit of this de-stressing can be better sleep.

these documents were convinced that lifestyle changes with an emphasis on relaxation could reverse the risk of heart attack, stroke, and stress symptoms like insomnia.

Benson outlined four essential elements necessary to elicit the positive physiological changes of the Relaxation Response: a quiet environment, a specific mental focus such as a repeated word, a passive and observing attitude, and a comfortable position.

Progressive Relaxation

Progressive Relaxation is another simple but powerful technique that can be practiced anywhere. It uses your own awareness of tension as a way to reduce it. Muscle relaxation and anxiety are incompatible. As you learn how to contract and release your muscles, you will experience an accompanying release of stress. This technique may be familiar to those who learned specific muscle-tensing and -relaxing techniques as preparation for childbirth.

Progressive Relaxation Instructions

Find a comfortable position, either lying down or sitting up. Beginning with your feet and progressing up your body, tense, then relax each muscle group. First, tighten your left foot, stretching it out as far as is comfortable. Hold the position for 5 seconds or so. Don't hold your breath. Now release. It is easier to experience the true relaxation of a muscle if you can contrast it to the feel of a tight one. Tense your foot one more time; hold for 5 seconds; release and relax. Do you notice any differences between your left foot and your right? You may sense a lightness, looseness, or warmth of the left foot. These are signs of muscle relaxation.

Try the same tightening and releasing on the calf, knee, and thigh muscles. Continue to tense and release. Alternate sides of your body. Move into the groin and stomach area, followed by your back and your arms and hands. End with your neck, face, and head. Really squeeze your eyes shut, hold, and then release. Do the same with your jaw muscles and your forehead.

10 Ways to a Better Night's Sleep

Many people who experience insomnia fail to alter their regular habits, convinced that some other factor is the cause of their problem. But often, the commonplace rituals we engage in every day are the source of sleep disturbances. Fortunately, there are a variety of simple ways to modify potentially harmful habits.

1. Create New Bedtime Rituals

Parents often create soothing bedtime rituals for their children. A bath followed by some cuddling in a rocking chair, a lullaby, or a story read aloud gives the evening an expected structure and allows little ones to slowly release the events and thoughts of the day. Adults also need this kind of release. What evening rituals would you find soothing, comforting, and relaxing? Doesn't a warm bath, some quiet time, light reading, a short phone call with a friend, or a cup of herbal tea sound good?

2. Don't Get Revved Up in the Evening

Not getting revved up in the evening means no suspenseful or scary stories. Try eliminating before-bed TV watching, and don't save that exciting best-seller for bedtime. Also, refrain from exercising within three hours of curfew.

3. Limit Caffeine

Coffee drinkers beware: Your habit may be hazardous to your sleep. Caffeine, alcohol, and cigarette smoking all decrease the quantity and quality of deep rest. Consuming 300 milligrams of caffeine — the equivalent of three cups of coffee or six cola drinks — at any time during a single day causes nighttime awakenings and disruption of the REM phase of sleep. Be aware that caffeine sensitivity can increase with age.

4. List Away Your Worries

The moment you place your head on the pillow is not the time to start thinking about all the things you have to do tomorrow, this week, or in your whole life. Instead, keep a list. At the end of your workday or before dinner, take 5 to 10 minutes to review the day's accomplishments and pleasures. Anything left undone, jot down.

Compile a list of 5 to 10 activities you plan to do tomorrow and rank them in order of importance. Add to this a master list or, as an on-line organizing forum suggests, a Mental Clutter List. Write down any idea or project that is on your mind, no matter how big or small. Break it down by the various roles in your life (employee, spouse, parent, community member, friend, and so forth) and by location (what has to be done in your house, in specific rooms of the house, in the garden, with the car, or the like).

Often people find that when they keep a list, they ruminate less before sleep and don't wake as often fretting about a remembered activity. If you wake up in the night feeling pressured by tasks that have to be done, write them down with paper and pen you keep on the nightstand.

5. Visualization: Remember Counting Sheep?

Have you heard the saying "Can't sleep, count sheep"? Although not currently a popular adage, this gem still has merit. If you truly visualize sheep one by one jumping over a white picket fence, all behind your eyelids, you've engaged your calm and creative center. Thinking and focusing on a repetitive image hardly leaves room for worries and other distracting concerns.

Another positive, calming exercise is to imagine a serene and private place. It may be on the shore of a lake, in a quiet and fragrant rose garden, out under the stars on a balmy summer night, or inside a cozy cabin deep in the pine woods; it may be a real or an imaginary place. Paint a picture in your mind using all five of your senses. What does your peaceful place look like, feel like, sound like, smell like? Is it warm and sunny, snug and luxurious, or coolly invigorating? Do not add other folks to this image. This place is yours and yours alone.

6. Approach Tomorrow Prepared and Refreshed

Sometimes it's hard to sleep the night before a big event. We anxiously await a job interview or a trip and then don't get the needed rest to positively meet the demands and pleasures ahead. Even daily tasks can create pressure. Take 15 to 30 minutes in the early evening to prepare for the next day's activities. Mental and physical preparation can range from carefully packing your suitcase to arranging your conference papers. On a daily basis, this may translate to making tomorrow's lunch or choosing clothes for yourself or young children.

7. Put the Fear Cycle to Sleep

"The only thing we have to fear is fear itself" is an apt description of the vicious cycle many of the sleep-deprived are victim to. Frantically, many an insomniac complains, "I just can't miss any more sleep." They focus on the fear and assume the worst, a phenomenon called catastrophizing.

Talking with a friend or a helping professional can assist you in regaining perspective: You will sleep again. When we are most pressured is when we can't sleep, so allow yourself options like the occasional late wake-up time, taking a day off from work or school, or canceling plans.

8. Establish a Regular Sleep Schedule

Many people with sleep problems think the way to handle their tiredness is to try to catch up on lost sleep during the weekends. Since the effect of missed sleep is cumulative, this technique can help only on a short-term basis. To conquer insomnia-related problems, it is best to go to bed at the same time every night and wake at the same time every morning, seven days a week.

9. Go to Bed Only When You Are Sleepy

This behavioral technique designed to conquer insomnia focuses on relearning how to associate going to bed with getting to sleep quickly and easily. In addition to cutting out afternoon naps and curbing reading or watching TV in bed, the Bootzin technique recommends that you get out of bed if you haven't fallen asleep within 10 minutes of getting into bed. If you wake during the night and can't go back to sleep, the same rule applies. Get back into bed only when you feel tired. If your insomnia is caused by a disrupted-sleep habit, this technique can help reinstill better sleep patterns.

10. Even If You Can't Sleep, Rest

Deepak Chopra disagrees with the Bootzin technique and other suggestions for getting up and occupying yourself when you are not sleeping. In *Restful Sleep*, Chopra recommends, "Rest with your eyes closed and let your awareness drift from sensation to sensation or thought to thought in a nonminding attitude. The more adept you become at using this technique, the better your sleep will be." He emphasizes the reparative process of rest.

Herbal Therapy

Herbs provide an extraordinary variety of aids for the sleepless. Aromatic herbal baths, compresses, and sleep pillows can lull you to sleep. And herbal teas and medicinal capsules, tinctures, and extracts are alternatives to over-the-counter and prescription sleep-inducing medications.

Why herbs? Many people are turning away from chemical sedatives and tranquilizers because of their side effects. Even when used as directed, these synthetic medicines can be habit forming, and many takers suffer a morning-after hangover. The products can also cause a distressing rebound effect, increasing the symptoms of anxiety and insomnia when they are discontinued.

An herbal renaissance has created an enormous increase in the use of natural remedies in the last few years, and the Europeans seem to be paving the way. In many European countries, herbal remedies are easily available in stores, and doctors' training focuses on complementary approaches to health issues. Prescriptions for herbal medicines are written by German physicians at a rate that equals that for American pharmaceuticals. Germany's Kommission E, a well-respected scientific committee, has issued reports attesting to the safety and efficacy of specific herbal remedies; physicians and consumers use this information in making treatment choices.

In the late 1990s, these monographs were translated into English to make this resource more accessible to North Americans. As another sign of the changing times, the large and somewhat daunting *Physician's Desk Reference* (known popularly as the *PDR*) — the standard reference book found in most medical offices that describes all available chemical prescription drugs — has recently issued an herbal medicine edition.

Using Herbs Safely

Herbs are a wonderful, all-natural remedy for sleeplessness. However, like all substances used for medicinal purposes,

Caution

- Do not take herbal sedatives or relaxants with alcohol, barbiturates, other sedatives, or other medications.
- Do not take strong sedatives if you are severely depressed.
- Do not take herbal sedatives while pregnant, except after consultation with your healthcare provider.
- Do not drive a car or operate machinery when taking an herbal sedative.
- Do not use any remedy nightly; there is a chance of building up a tolerance or dependence.

herbs must be administered with caution to be both safe and effective. When you use herbs, here are some ideas to keep in mind.

• The goal is to achieve unmedicated sleep. Herbal remedies, especially internal ones, are only for short-term use.

• Just because herbs are natural doesn't mean you don't have to follow precautions when taking them. Follow recommended doses; more is not better.

• Start with the gentler herbs and remedies, like a cup of chamomile tea and an herbal bath, before moving on to the stronger remedies.

• If you are currently taking medications for insomnia, do not stop abruptly. A healthcare practitioner can help you adjust the dosages so that the weaning process doesn't cause side effects.

• Read about the remedies and lifestyle changes you are anticipating. Join or start a support group.

10 Herbs for Sleep and Relaxation

There are many herbs renowned for their sleep-inducing and relaxing qualities. The choices include herbs that are primarily used internally in the form of medicinal teas, capsules, and tinctures. Others are more often used in herbal bath formulas and sleep pillows. All of the herbs mentioned here are readily available at healthfood stores or through mail order.

10 Herbs and Their Uses

Since most of the herbs can be used in multiple forms, the chart accents their primary use.

Herb	Characteristics	Form	Primary use
Catnip	Mild sedative	Tea	For occasional sleeplessness
Chamomile	Mild sedative	Tea	Relaxing; also good for stomachaches
Hops	Moderate strength, bitter tasting	Tea, dried, tincture	In sleep pillows
Kava-kava	Moderate strength, bitter tasting	Tincture, capsules	To relieve anxiety, muscle tension
Lavender	Sedative, aromatic	Dried, essential oil	For relaxing sleep-inducing baths and compresses; also good for headache relief
Lemon balm	Moderate strength, good taste	Tea, tincture	Relaxing and calming for sleeplessness
Oat straw	Mild	Tea, tincture	To relieve nervousness and insomnia
Passion-flower	Moderate strength	Tincture, capsule	Sedative, good in combinations
Skullcap	Moderate strength	Tea, tincture	Relaxing; also good for tension headaches
Valerian	Strong sedative, bad odor	Tincture, capsules	Excellent sleep inducer; also for cramps

Catnip (*Nepeta cataria*)

Did you know that catnip has opposite effects in people and cats? What stimulates cats in stuffed toys and teases them in the garden is regarded as a mild sedative for humans. Fresh or dried catnip, a cousin to mint, makes a nice tea. Because I grow my own and have extra after bottling my harvest for winter beverages, I add catnip to both my bath and sleep-pillow formulas.

Chamomile (*Matricaria recutita*)

Chamomile's pretty white flowers with yellow centers make a lovely mild, relaxing tea and are good in baths for sleepless adults and fussy babies. Peter Rabbit's mother served him a cup of chamomile after his escape from Mr. McGregor's garden. Many herbalists also recommend this gentle herb as a colic remedy for children. Chamomile has a relaxing effect on the nervous and digestive systems and has anti-inflammatory effects. It is included on the list of herbs that the FDA deems "generally regarded as safe."

In addition to being a sleep aid, chamomile has traditionally been used to treat stomachaches, ulcers, menstrual cramps, and arthritis. Internal and external remedies use the plant's healing qualities. It is purported to both prevent infection and serve as an immune system stimulant. Chamomile has also been used to heal wounds. Compresses and baths made with infused flowers soothe irritated and inflamed skin.

Although I often recommend infusing medicinal teas for a longer period of time, if you desire a mild, pleasant-tasting tea, don't steep chamomile for more than 10 minutes; it becomes more bitter the longer it is steeped. You can brew it alone or in combination with other sedating herbs.

This herb is a major ingredient in many commercial tea blends, like Celestial Seasonings Sleepytime Tea.

On its own, chamomile may be too weak a sleep promoter for adults. Many find it slightly calming, a nice break during a busy day. The lovely bath book *Water Magic* by Mary Muryn and Cathy Cash Spellman (Fireside, 1995) describes a chamomile immersion for a Sleep-Like-a-Baby-Bath. Following a chamomile facial steam, wet chamomile tea bags are put over your closed eyes while you lie in a tub of chamomile-infused waters and sip a steaming cup of chamomile tea. Accompanied by a scented candle, soothing music, and an aromatic sleep pillow scented with chamomile, almost any adult could be lulled to sleep. (Wait until you are out of the bath and comfortably in bed!)

As with all herb use, individual reactions may differ. Some people can have an allergic reaction to chamomile, especially those who suffer from hay fever or other ragweed allergies.

Hops (*Humulus lupulus*)

The strongly scented, conelike flowers of the hop plant can be used externally or internally for inducing sleep. It is common knowledge that hops are used in beermaking, but initially they were not favored as an additive to beer and ale because they turned the formerly sweet-tasting ale bitter.

Historically, Chinese physicians used hops to treat leprosy, tuberculosis, and dysentery. The plant was cultivated in Roman gardens; the young shoots were eaten as a vegetable. But hop farmers observed a most noteworthy effect: Those who harvested the perennial climbing plants suffered symptoms of fatigue. Native Americans used them for their sedative and digestion-aiding properties. An old Pennsylvania Dutch remedy for headache or toothache pain called for having the victim lie on a clean sock filled with warmed hops.

Hops are considered stronger than chamomile as a remedy for insomnia. Perhaps hops haven't reached chamomile's popularity because of their somewhat bitter taste. Hops should be used in a dried, aged form. The plant loses its effectiveness rapidly when stored, so buy small amounts. The FDA includes hops on its list of herbs "generally regarded as safe."

Hops have estrogenic properties; their effects in the body are similar to those of female hormones. Thus, hops should not be used in formulas taken by breast cancer patients. The hormonal effect seems to have advantages for menopausal women, however. Herbalist Susun Weed recommends hop tea as a powerful sleep enhancer and hormonal ally to women frequently awakened by night sweats.

The sedative qualities of hops are best experienced when used in teas, in tincture combinations, externally in baths, and as a major ingredient in sleep pillows.

Kava-Kava *(Piper methysticum)*

Kava-kava is a wonderful herbal remedy for mild to moderate anxiety. Studies also indicate that it may be an effective treatment for insomnia.

Kava-kava's popularity and usage have recently increased in the United States. It is touted as an all-natural antianxiety treatment with fewer side effects than prescription medications. Kava-kava produces a pleasant sense of relaxation and a sharpening of the senses while maintaining mental alertness; pharmaceutical antianxiety medications are more sedating, and they slow down many mental and physical functions. In addition, kava-kava, unlike its pharmaceutical counterparts, does not cause physical addiction or withdrawal symptoms when taken in recommended doses. There have been a few reports of serious side effects ranging from skin disorders to dependence, but only with very high doses over a long period of time.

A visit to the natural-food and supplement store will provide you with a range of kava-kava products. It is available in teas, capsules, extracts, and in a dried, powdered form. Be forewarned: Kava-kava is another bitter-tasting herb. When the powder is mixed with water, the resulting drink has been likened to Novocain in both taste and function: Because of its analgesic properties, drinking kava-kava does numb the mouth.

Kava-kava produces relaxation without sedation, making it a good choice to counter daytime stress and anxiety. A German study attested to the herb's ability to alleviate anxiety associated with menopause.

Anecdotal accounts of kava-kava's worth as a sleep aid vary. Some people report that since the herb increases alertness, it can interfere with the ability to fall asleep. It seems that the size and timing of the dose may affect its sleep-enhancing properties. After the initial alertness wears off, subsequent sleep can be deep and refreshing. A small dose taken earlier during the day may produce alertness, relaxation, and, later, sleep.

Lavender (*Lavandula officinalis, L. vera,* and *L. angustifolia* subsp. *angustifolia*)

The beauty of its deep color as well as its highly evocative scent have made lavender a favorite for many centuries. It is a safe and simple sedative when used in baths, massage oils, compresses, aromatherapy diffusers, and sleep pillows. Some herbalists also add it to various relaxing tea blends. Versatile lavender has been included as an ingredient in the Egyptian mummification process and used as a wound healer in World War I; it was a favorite of English royalty for their gardens, teas, and linens.

Most of us are familiar with lavender's fragrance in a multitude of laundry products and toiletries. In addition to appearing in a wonderful variety of soaps, lotions, and oils, lavender is a top choice for potpourris, wreaths, and sachets. The French have given the dried, deep blue-violet flowers a culinary role as a major ingredient in herbes de Provence, an herb mix used to flavor soups and stews. Adventurous cooks add lavender flowers or leaves to flavor teas, cookies, cakes, and fruit salads. Vinegar infused with lavender and a hint of mint can be found in the kitchen to enhance desserts, or even in the bath for a face wash.

Lavender has a long-standing reputation for medicinal qualities. External applications help combat insomnia, tension, and headaches. It is purported to have antispasmodic, analgesic, antidepressant, antiseptic, sedative, and other healing qualities. Lavender has been used to soothe wounds, burns, and irritated skin conditions. Current studies are investigating its possible cancer-fighting components, since it's been shown to reduce the size of breast cancer tumors in mice.

Pretty impressive. And yet lavender is easy to use right in your own home. I suggest incorporating the dried or fresh flowers or the essential oil into external-use sleep aids. Alone or mixed with complementary herbs and flowers, lavender makes a great bath additive. It also is a major ingredient in my favorite sleep pillow; resting your head on a pillow filled with lavender releases the wonderful relaxing aroma and helps promote a wonderfully restoring night's sleep.

Lemon Balm *(Melissa officinalis)*
The luscious citrus taste and aroma of lemon balm are sedating and good for stomachaches. Historically, lemon balm has been used to treat headaches, menstrual cramps, and wounds as well as

nervousness and anxiety. In studies that used a combination of valerian extract and lemon balm, the effects were shown to be as powerful as those of pharmaceutical sleep medications. And the sweet, citrusy lemon balm masks the unpleasant valerian flavor.

Michael Castleman, author of *Healing Herbs: The Ultimate Guide to the Curative Power of Nature's Medicines,* cautions that since lemon balm can interfere with a thyroid-stimulating hormone, those who have thyroid problems should consult their physicians before using it.

Lemon balm is wonderfully versatile. Use it as a great-tasting and relaxing tea or tincture, or add it to bath and sleep-pillow mixes.

Oat Straw (*Avena sativa*)

A cup of oat straw tea? More familiar, of course, is our eating of the traditional nourishing breakfast oatmeal. But herbalists Susun Weed and Deb Soule recommend oat straw tea as a gentle, soothing, and nourishing relaxant. Oats are thought to strengthen the nervous system and relieve pain. In the bath, oats soothe irritated skin.

Although it may not be strong enough for those with persistent sleep problems, a warm cup of oat straw tea with milk may relieve the occasional sleepless night caused by nervous tension, anxiety, or menopausal symptoms.

Passionflower (*Passiflora incarnata*)

Herbalists believe that passionflower has been a favored sleep remedy since the days of the Aztecs and Incas. It is still widely used in Brazil to treat insomnia, anxiety, and nervousness.

Passionflower combines well with valerian and is often used as a supplement in tea, capsule, and tincture forms. Passionflower tea can be enjoyed throughout the day, but for refreshing sleep, drink the tea or take the tincture half an hour before bedtime.

Skullcap (*Scutellaria lateriflora*)

Herbalists have much anecdotal evidence as to the merits of skullcap as a relaxant and sedative. Skullcap is the herb of choice for treating all nervous disorders, including stress and insomnia. It has also been used as an antispasmodic, treating muscle cramps and spasms.

The recommended use of skullcap is as a tea or tincture. Viewed as a wonderful supplement to stronger herbal sedatives, skullcap is often included in commercial combination formulas.

Valerian (*Valeriana officinalis*)

Valerian is the herb of choice for insomnia and stress. It also works well for reducing menstrual cramps, headaches associated with the menstrual cycle, and intestinal upsets. The FDA places it on its list of herbs "generally regarded as safe."

German studies have substantiated valerian's benefits as a relaxant without sedative side effects. Those who take it at night have been rewarded with deep sleep, awakening refreshed in the morning. Valerian eliminates the morning-after grogginess associated with chemical tranquilizers. Herbalists recommend valerian as a nonaddictive and non-habit-forming remedy.

Like many herbal remedies, valerian has a proud history of use. The famous 12th-century German abbess and herbalist Hildegard of Bingen recommended valerian as a tranquilizer and sleep aid. Europeans also included valerian in formulas to treat conditions from the plague to epilepsy. And supposedly it was the hypnotic employed by the Pied Piper of Hamelin to rid the town of rats.

So what are valerian's drawbacks? Most notably, it has a strong, unpleasant odor.

My family always knows when I've opened the jar of dried valerian root — the house smells like a locker room full of dirty socks. To overcome this real aesthetic disadvantage, I recommend taking valerian in its more palatable forms, as either a capsule or a tincture. Although the strong taste is still evident in the tincture, this form may be chosen for its strength. A combination formula, especially one with the sedative and pleasant-tasting lemon balm, is a good alternative.

Another problem with valerian is that in a small percentage of takers, it causes the opposite effect of what is desired: It is stimulating rather than relaxing. However, these symptoms immediately disappear when the herb is discontinued.

The recommended dose of valerian, as with other sedative herbs, depends on the form and brand that you are taking. Many herbalists recommend a dropperful of the tincture in some water at bedtime. More than one practitioner tells stories of clients complaining that valerian wasn't helpful to them. This may simply be due to starting with too small a dose. If the recommended amount doesn't work for you or if you have been taking prescription drugs, talk to your healthcare practitioner about how to adjust your intake.

How to Use Herbs for Sleep

Despite the fancy names and technical terms, using herbs in formulas for relaxation is quite simple. You won't need much in the way of equipment, supplies, or time — just an open mind and the desire to achieve health-giving, quality sleep.

Herbal Teas

Feeling stressed? Forget the coffee break. Instead, brew yourself a cup of relaxing, noncaffeinated chamomile or catnip tea. Having trouble sleeping? Add a cup of sedating tea to your evening ritual. Commercial blends with names like Sleepytime, Tran-kwil, and SereniTea are available on the grocery and health-food-store shelves.

Herbal Tinctures and Extracts

When a more potent herbal sleep aid is needed, you can take a liquid herbal formula. Dr. Andrew Weil recommends tinctures and freeze-dried extracts of medicinal plants as your best purchases. Tinctures and extracts are convenient, stable, and usually standardized. An alcohol base is common, because it extracts and preserves the most useful plant constituents. For those sensitive to alcohol, there are glycerin-based alternatives.

Extracts of a combination of sedative herbs like valerian, lemon balm, passionflower, and chamomile are available as an aid for temporary insomnia. Kava-kava tincture may be more useful to relieve anxiety and muscle tension.

Herbal Baths

Not feeling sleepy tonight? Take a bath. Baths feel wonderful and are powerful sleep inducers. There is a correlation between body temperature and sleep; we get sleepy when our body temperatures naturally drop in the evening. That drop is assisted when we cool off after a bath.

Add herbs to a bath and you've got one of the best natural sleep remedies there is. The body physically responds to the different chemicals emitted by flowers, and some specific scents — including lavender, chamomile, rose, and hops — are sedating. There are many ways to enjoy herbal baths. My favorites include bath salts, bath bags, and herbal infusions for the tub.

Bath salts can be purchased, or you can make them yourself at home. Simple homemade versions usually include a combination of sea salt and Epsom salts with a baking soda base. Then add the fragrant and relaxing scent of an individual essential oil or a mix of oils. Pour in the prepared salts while the bathtub is filling; as they dissolve, they emit a lovely aroma.

Sleepy-Time Bath Salts

This recipe can be easily increased. I often make batches of 6 cups at a time. Remember, you want the scent to be strong; it will be diluted in the bath.

⅓ cup sea salt
⅓ cup Epsom salts
⅓ cup baking soda
7 drops chamomile essential oil
4 drops lavender essential oil
4 drops marjoram essential oil
5 drops food coloring of choice (optional)
¼ teaspoon glycerin (optional)

1. Mix the dry ingredients together in a medium-size bowl. Use a metal, ceramic, or other nonporous container; do not use plastic. Add the essential oils and stir. If desired, add food coloring and glycerin and mix until well blended.

2. Cover the bowl with a cotton cloth and leave to dry overnight. Stir again, breaking up any small chunks, before pouring into containers.

3. To use: Pour ½ cup into the tub as it is filling.

Essential oils are concentrated essences of naturally occurring oils from plants and flowers. They are commercially distilled or extracted and used in perfumery and aromatherapy. For a full discussion of their uses, see *The Essential Oils Book* by Colleen Dodt (Storey Books, 1996). If you don't want to purchase a number of essential oils, you may want to buy premade bath salts. The popularity of bath products has increased in the last few years, and various salts are now available.

Infusions

Herbal infusions are strong teas. The selected herbs are placed in a pan or jar, covered with boiling water, and left to steep for a minimum of 15 minutes. Obviously, the longer you steep the herbs, the more concentrated the solution will be. The container needs to be covered so that the strong fragrance will not be lost. Then the highly aromatic, strained herbal tea is poured into the bath as it is being filled.

Insomniac's Bath Infusion

Choose one or more of the following herbs: chamomile, catnip, lavender, lemon balm, passionflower, or rose petals. If desired, add a small amount of hops or valerian root.

    1–2 cups fresh or dried herbs of choice
       1 quart boiling water

Place the herbs in a jar. Cover with boiling water and steep for at least 15 minutes. When done, strain the mixture through a mesh strainer or a colander covered with cheese-cloth. Pour the fluid into the bath as it is being drawn.

Herbal Bath Bags

Herbal bath bags are another convenient way to immerse yourself in herbal pleasure. The bags are made by placing a fresh or dried herb combination in the middle of a fabric square and tying it closed. This is essentially like making a large tea bag to brew in a very large "teacup" — your bathtub. A major advantage of this method is that there are no loose flowers to clean out of the tub. And since these aromatic treats are generally made ahead of time, preparation and planning time are limited.

Oatmeal and dried milk can be combined with herbs and flowers to add other soothing qualities to the sedating scents. Washcloths, small cotton drawstring bags, and fancy old cloth handkerchiefs all make attractive, easy wrappings. Hang the sachet from the bathtub faucet and let the water run through the herbs. The tie can be colorfast string or ribbon.

Be sure to experiment. The most sedating, soothing bath for you will be one that you spontaneously and positively react to. If you think "Oh, that smells great," or "Phew, that smells awful," go with your attraction. Don't use a formula you don't like just because it's supposed to be relaxing. The exceptions to the rule are valerian and hops, whose fragrance many people do not like. Try them first in small amounts. And don't make your final judgment until you have added all the more-fragrant herbs.

Blissful Sleep Bath Bags

I love a lemon-scented bath; the lemon balm, hops, and catnip are great sedative herbs, and the calendula is a gentle skin soother. The orange peel adds a sweet and joyful note to the mixture.

1 cup dried calendula petals
1 cup dried lemon balm
½ cup dried hops
½ cup dried catnip
A few pieces of dried orange peel (optional)

Combine all ingredients. Place ½ cup of the mixture in the middle of a piece of permeable fabric and tie closed. When running the bath, loop the tie over the faucet so the water runs through the bag as the tub fills.

Soothing Smoothing Bath Bags

Especially great in the wintertime, this recipe includes oats and milk to create an insomnia-abating bath with additional skin-soothing properties.

1 cup oatmeal
½ cup dried milk powder
1 cup dried rose petals
1 cup dried lavender flowers
½ cup dried lemon verbena
¼ cup dried rosemary

Combine all ingredients. Place ½ cup of the mixture in the middle of a piece of permeable fabric and tie closed. When running the bath, loop the tie over the faucet so the water runs through the bag as the tub fills.

Calming Waters Bath Bags

I love the evocative scent of lavender. Here it is complemented by other pleasantly scented, sleep-promoting herbs. Valerian doesn't have a pleasant scent, but it is very soothing, and the other herbs counteract its smell.

2 cups dried lavender flowers
1 cup dried chamomile flowers
½ cup dried hops flowers
½ cup dried passionflower
¼ cup dried valerian root (optional)

Combine all ingredients. Place ½ cup of the mixture in the middle of a piece of permeable fabric and tie closed. When running the bath, loop the tie over the faucet so the water runs through the bag as the tub fills.

Herbal Compresses

Feeling stressed and hoping for some physical comfort, but don't have time for a bath? Take five and try a comforting, aromatic herbal compress. To make one, add a handful of fresh or dried lavender flowers, chamomile, or lemon balm to a bowl of hot water. Saturate a washcloth or other clean cloth in the warm water, squeeze out the excess, and apply it to your neck or forehead. Lie down and close your eyes. If you have a headache, use lavender flowers or lavender essential oil for the compress.

Sleep Pillows

I was introduced to dream pillows at a workshop given by one of my favorite herbalists, Susun Weed, at her home in Woodstock, New York. On a warm and sunny spring afternoon, a group of us sat on Susun's back deck, where she had assembled a large assortment of fabrics and bags of herbs. We passed around the containers full of exotic-sounding and distinctively aromatic plants: mugwort, hops, lavender, mint, basil, rosemary, sage, oregano, chamomile, rosebuds, and red clover. Each workshop participant hand-stitched a fabric envelope and filled the form with an individualized mixture while Susun explained the various attributes of each herb. Later in the day, we had a show-and-tell session to share our creations. Each pillow looked and smelled different.

When I returned home, I learned that sleep pillows have a long history. For example, Phyllis V. Shaudys, in her book *The Pleasure of Herbs* (Storey Books, 1986), reports that herbal pillows or "sleep bags" were used in colonial times to induce sleep and healing for the sick.

The practical concerns when making herbal pillows are the size and shape of the pillow, the fabric it is covered with and its ability to be cleaned, and the choice of herbs and other fillings. A small pillow that is flat, not plump, is recommended. You can place it in between your usual pillow and pillowcase. Its sweet, calming smell will be released each time you squeeze it or turn your head on it. Pillow sizes usually range from a small 4-inch square to a fuller 11 by 9 inches.

There are many great fabric textures, weights, and designs to choose from. Some sewers prefer calico, chintz, or a soft, light flannel. Fabrics with a celestial pattern that match the evening dream theme are available. For durability, you can make an inner muslin pillow filled with herbs, then cover this pouch with a detachable and washable cover. I keep a basket of small, fragrant sleep pillows, all covered with different fabrics, in the hall outside the guest room. A friend who owns a bed-and-breakfast keeps optional scented pillows around for her herbally minded patrons.

Obviously, the most important consideration in filling an herbal sleep pillow is choosing the right combination of sedating scents to help the recipient relax and sleep. Lavender, chamomile, lemon balm, hops, and roses are

Nighty-Night Dream-Pillow Mix

This recipe combines all my favorite sleep-pillow herbs. Adjust the proportions based on personal preference and availability.

- 4 parts dried lavender flowers
- 2 parts dried rose petals
- 2 parts dried hops
- 1 part dried chamomile
- 1 part dried lemon balm

some pleasing soporific herbs to start with. Jim Long provides a number of recipes for dream and sleep pillows in his book *Making Herbal Dream Pillows* (Storey Books, 1998).

Not all relaxing herbs have pleasant aromas or associations for the sleeper. For example, many find hops too bitter-smelling. But combined with sweeter-scented herbs like lavender and rose, hops increase the sleep-inducing properties of the pillow while its smell is toned down.

Some books recommend making pillow blends as if they were potpourri, but I have found that the best sleep-pillow mixtures leave out certain potpourri ingredients. Preservatives like orrisroot can cause allergic reactions, and essential oils create a very powerful scent.

Finally, you can fill your pillow with herbs alone or shape it first with cotton batting or a synthetic pillow stuffing like Fiberfill. It is generally cheaper to make pillows with this type of filler. Sprinkle 1 to 2 tablespoons of herb mix between thin layers of the stuffing. This method also ensures a softer pillow, lessening the chance of leaves or twigs sticking through the pillow cover.

Sleep Pillows for Children

Pillows recommended as sleep aids for children are often filled with one herb — usually dill, chamomile, or catnip. These three herbs are purported to gently lull a child to sleep and to deter nightmares. A soft, multilayered flannel pillow is a cozy comfort. Presents of homemade stuffed animals or rag dolls filled with soothing herb mixtures and named Dreaming Darlene and Sleepy Sam are much appreciated. For a store-bought alternative, try the Sleep Bunny, a wonderfully soft and cuddly herb-filled sleep partner.

And Now, Good Night

As you have read, there are many alternatives to sleepless nights. First, accurately assess your sleep problem using the sleep diary questions, and then contact professional helpers if necessary. Experiment with one or more of the various self-help strategies and you can regain a refreshing, healthy sleep pattern.

Good luck, good health, and good sleep!